TINNITUS DIET FOR NEWLY DIAGNOSED

Discover Nutritional Solutions, Proven Strategies, Meal Plans, Medical Insights, And Lifestyle Tips To Manage Tinnitus And Regain Serenity

DR. ERIC TRISTAN

CONTENTS

DISCLAIMER

The information provided in this book, is intended for informational purposes only. The content is not intended to be a substitute for professional medical advice, diagnosis, or treatment. Always seek the advice of your physician or other qualified health provider with any questions you may have regarding a medical condition. Never disregard professional medical advice or delay in seeking it because of something you have read in this book.

The author of this book has made reasonable efforts to ensure that the information provided is accurate and up-to-date at the time of publication. However, the author makes no representations or warranties of any kind, express or implied, about the completeness, accuracy, reliability, suitability, or availability of the information contained within these pages.

Any reliance you place on the information provided in this book is strictly at your own risk. The author shall not be liable for any loss, injury, or damage arising from the use of this book or the information contained herein.

The mention or reference to any individuals, products, websites, organizations, or other names within this book does not imply endorsement by the author. The inclusion of such references is solely for informational purposes and does not constitute an endorsement or recommendation.

Furthermore, the author disclaims any association or affiliation with any individuals, products, websites, organizations, or other names mentioned in this book.

It is important to consult with a qualified healthcare professional before making any dietary or lifestyle changes, especially if you have a medical condition. Each individual's health situation is unique, and what works for one person may not work for another.

Again, the information provided in this book is not intended to diagnose, treat, cure, or prevent any disease or health condition. Always seek the advice of a physician or other qualified health provider regarding any medical questions or concerns you may have.

Thank you for your understanding and for taking the necessary precautions when considering the information presented in this book.

ABOUT THIS BOOK

This book entitled "Tinnitus Diet" presents an extensive and perceptive analysis of the critical correlation between diet and tinnitus, thereby furnishing invaluable recommendations for those who wish to effectively cope with this frequently difficult ailment. The introductory segment establishes the groundwork by providing a comprehensive overview of tinnitus, guaranteeing that readers comprehend its complex and varied characteristics. Subsequently, this book explores the complex relationship between diet and tinnitus, placing particular emphasis on the crucial impact that nutrition has on the origins of tinnitus.

The table of contents provides a comprehensive breakdown of the intricate topic, covering different aspects of dietary selections and their influence on tinnitus. In addition to a curated list of foods that are sympathetic to tinnitus, the reader acquires a profound comprehension of particular foods that ought to be avoided.

This book emphasizes the holistic approach to managing tinnitus through the incorporation of lifestyle modifications, nutritional supplements, and hydration as essential elements of the discourse.

Moreover, this book delves into the intricate correlation that exists between tinnitus and everyday substances including caffeine, alcohol, sodium, sugar, and gluten. An examination of the Mediterranean diet imbues dietary practices that potentially exert a beneficial impact on tinnitus with a cultural dimension. The pragmatic nature of the book's suggestions in real-world situations is emphasized by the incorporation of personalized diet plans and guidance on progress monitoring.

This book's emphasis on the importance of consulting professionals is an especially praiseworthy element. This highlights the significance of personalized attention and recognizes the distinct characteristics of every individual's tinnitus experience.

Ultimately, "Tinnitus Diet" serves as a highly beneficial resource for individuals contending with tinnitus, providing an all-encompassing manual that skillfully integrates pragmatic suggestions for dietary and lifestyle adjustments with scientifically grounded advice.

CHAPTER ONE

An Overview Of The Tinnitus Diet

Constantly manifesting as a ringing, humming, or hissing sensation in the hearing, tinnitus is a difficult condition that impacts millions of individuals across the globe. Although a definitive cure for tinnitus has yet to be discovered, the importance of incorporating a balanced diet into one's healthy lifestyle has gained recognition as a critical component in symptom management. This investigation examines the complex correlation between tinnitus and diet, specifically investigating the potential influence of dietary choices on the frequency and intensity of tinnitus.

Comprehension Of Tinnitus

Tinnitus is a symptom of an underlying condition, frequently associated with injury to the auditory system and not a disease. Exposure to harsh sounds, age-related hearing loss, earwax blockages, or even specific medications may cause this injury. Individuals who suffer from tinnitus may endure distressing and persistent spectral sounds, which hurt their overall quality of life. It is critical to comprehend the underlying mechanisms of tinnitus to formulate efficacious management strategies.

Tinnitus occurs when the brain receives signals from the auditory nerves that produce the sensation of sound in the absence of an external stimulus. A variety of factors, such as diet, stress, and anxiety, can affect this aberrant signaling. Although tinnitus symptoms can be triggered or worsened by stress and anxiety, there is a growing body of research that examines the potential influence of dietary choices on auditory health.

Dietary Influence On Tinnitus

Emerging evidence indicates that in addition to its critical impact on overall health, diet may also affect tinnitus. An antioxidant, vitamin, and mineral-rich diet is beneficial to the health of the auditory system. Fruits and vegetables contain antioxidants, which aid in the fight against oxidative stress, a factor in numerous health conditions, including hearing disorders.

By prioritizing whole foods in one's diet, cardiovascular health can be enhanced and the likelihood of developing conditions such as atherosclerosis, which can obstruct blood flow to the ears, is decreased. Ensuring adequate blood flow is critical for the preservation of the inner ear's functionality, which houses the auditory system.

Fish, flaxseeds, and walnuts contain omega-3 fatty acids, which possess anti-inflammatory properties that might be advantageous for those who suffer from tinnitus. Intestinal inflammation may potentially exacerbate symptoms of tinnitus; therefore, a diet rich in omega-3 fatty acids may be beneficial in reducing this inflammation.

Conversely, an excessive intake of processed foods, saturated lipids, and sugar may negatively impact the management of tinnitus. The consumption of these dietary options may potentially exacerbate tinnitus symptoms by promoting inflammation, elevating oxidative stress, and impeding blood flow. In light of ongoing scientific inquiry into the correlation between tinnitus and diet, it seems prudent to consider implementing a nutritious and well-balanced diet as a potential strategy for managing this condition.

Anti-Tinnitus Factors

Diet, similar to other environmental and lifestyle factors, can catalyze tinnitus. Common ingredients in many diets, caffeine, and nicotine are recognized stimulants that can worsen the symptoms of tinnitus. Elevated heart rate and blood pressure may result from the use of these substances, which may exacerbate the sensation of tinnitus.

Additionally, a high sodium intake is a dietary component associated with tinnitus. Elevated concentrations of sodium have the potential to induce fluid retention and influence blood pressure, both of which may have adverse effects on the fragile structures of the inner ear. Individuals predisposed to tinnitus may experience symptomatic relief by decreasing their sodium consumption.

Additionally, alcohol consumption may impact tinnitus. Although moderate alcohol consumption may not present substantial complications, excessive drinking has the potential to aggravate tinnitus symptoms by causing dehydration and interfering with blood circulation. Tinnitus sufferers may benefit from the practice of monitoring and regulating their alcohol consumption.

Items To Prevent

Certain food items may be contemplated as alternatives to alleviate the symptoms of tinnitus. Restricting consumption of salty munchies, processed foods, and those high in refined carbohydrates is advisable due to their potential to promote inflammation and undermine general well-being. Furthermore, reducing one's consumption of caffeine, nicotine, and alcohol may assist in alleviating the stimuli that cause tinnitus.

Unnatural sweeteners are an additional possible offender. Although there is a scarcity of research examining the direct effects of artificial sweeteners on tinnitus, certain individuals have reported a correlation between their use of such products and an exacerbation of tinnitus symptoms. Individuals experiencing tinnitus must vigilantly monitor their reaction to these additives and make well-informed dietary decisions to experience relief.

In summary, although there is no universally applicable strategy for dietary management of tinnitus, incorporating a balanced and nutritious diet into one's routine could potentially improve overall health and mitigate certain symptoms. A comprehensive comprehension of the complex correlation between diet and tinnitus enables individuals to exercise agency over their health and quality of life by enabling them to make well-informed decisions. As further investigations reveal the intricacies of this correlation, maintaining a healthy dietary regimen continues to be a prudent and proactive course of action for individuals grappling with the difficulties associated with tinnitus.

Otitis Neuritis-Friendly Foods: Ear-Soothing Sounds

A persistent ringing, humming, or hissing sound in the hearing constitutes tinnitus, which can be a difficult condition to control. Although medical treatments are available, individuals are increasingly considering the adoption of a tinnitus-friendly diet as a potential method to alleviate symptoms. The inclusion of particular dietary items recognized for their potential health benefits could potentially enhance the comfort level of individuals who are afflicted with tinnitus.

Specific dietary nutrients and compounds may contribute to the alleviation of tinnitus symptoms. Berry, spinach, and kale are examples of antioxidant-rich foods that may aid in the fight against oxidative stress, a process thought to be associated with tinnitus. The omega-3 fatty acids present in fatty fish such as mackerel and salmon may possess beneficial anti-inflammatory properties.

It is vital to maintain stable blood sugar levels to effectively manage tinnitus. By selecting whole grains, lean proteins, and low-glycemic fruits, individuals may potentially mitigate the severity of tinnitus symptoms by aiding in blood sugar regulation. Furthermore, the consumption of foods abundant in magnesium, such as bananas, almonds, and leafy greens, may prove advantageous due to the hypothesis that magnesium influences neuronal function.

Although a universally applicable tinnitus-friendly diet does not exist, certain individuals have reported favorable outcomes by abstaining from specific trigger foods. These may consist of alcohol, stimulants, and high-sodium foods. For some individuals, these substances may be more effectively managed as tinnitus symptoms are avoided or their consumption is restricted.

CHAPTER TWO

Supplemental Nutrition For Tinnitus: Bridging The Relief Gap

Alongside the implementation of a tinnitus-friendly diet, the inclusion of nutritional supplements in a comprehensive regimen for symptom management can prove to be beneficial. The purpose of these nutritional supplements is to augment the body's nutrition with specific nutrients that are critical for maintaining optimal ear health and well-being.

Ginkgo biloba, a supplement frequently investigated for its purported antioxidant and vasodilatory properties, is one such substance. Ginkgo biloba may enhance blood flow to the ears and alleviate tinnitus symptoms, according to some studies. Before adding any supplement to your routine, it is vital to consult a healthcare professional, as individual responses may vary.

Vitamin B12 is an additional nutrient associated with tinnitus. Neurological issues can result from B12 deficiency; therefore, supplementation may be beneficial for those who experience tinnitus associated with such deficiencies. Although vitamin B12 is naturally present in animal products such as meat, fish, and dairy, individuals with dietary restrictions or absorption issues may benefit from supplementation.

Zinc, a vital mineral, is essential for wound healing and the functioning of the immune system. Zinc supplementation may alleviate the symptoms of tinnitus, particularly in individuals with insufficient zinc levels, according to some studies. However, excessive zinc consumption can result in negative side effects; therefore, it is imperative to adhere to recommended guidelines and seek guidance from a healthcare professional.

Tinnitus And Hydration: Alleviating The Ringing

Maintaining sufficient fluid intake is critical for optimal physiological functioning and could potentially contribute to the alleviation of tinnitus symptoms. Alterations in blood circulation caused by dehydration may impact the inner ear and potentially exacerbate tinnitus.

Adequate hydration throughout the day aids in the maintenance of healthy blood circulation and viscosity. Enhanced perfusion has the potential to exert a beneficial influence on tinnitus symptoms by potentially mitigating the severity of the condition's functional manifestations. Although hydration in isolation may not provide a cure for tinnitus, it is a straightforward and readily available modification to one's way of life that can be integrated into the daily schedule.

It is imperative to restrict the consumption of dehydrating substances, including alcohol and caffeine. Both substances have the potential to cause dehydration, which may worsen the symptoms of tinnitus.

Selecting hydrating alternatives, such as infused water or herbal beverages, can be a tasty and tinnitus-friendly method to maintain adequate hydration.

Modifications To One's Lifestyle To Manage Tinnitus: Beyond The Ringing

Certain modifications to one's lifestyle, in conjunction with dietary adjustments and nutritional supplements, have the potential to enhance the overall quality of life for individuals afflicted with tinnitus. Critical is the management of tension, as it can exacerbate tinnitus symptoms. The integration of relaxation modalities, including yoga, meditation, and deep breathing, may prove advantageous in the mitigation of stress levels.

Additionally, noise management is a crucial component of tinnitus lifestyle adjustments. White noise devices or calming background sounds are frequently utilized by those with tinnitus to disguise the ringing or buzzing. Additionally, ear protection can aid in the management of tinnitus symptoms and prevent further auditory harm by being worn in noisy environments.

Physical activity regularly has been associated with general health and may indirectly benefit those with tinnitus. Physical activity enhances circulation, alleviates tension, and facilitates restful slumber, all of which have the potential to positively impact the management of tinnitus. Participating in physical activities such as cycling, strolling, or swimming can provide pleasure and support an individual's way of life.

In summary, although there is no universally applicable remedy for tinnitus management, some individuals may find respite through a combination of a dietary regimen tailored to tinnitus, nutritional supplements, adequate hydration, and adjustments to their lifestyle. It is imperative to seek guidance from healthcare professionals before implementing substantial dietary or supplement modifications, as individual reactions to these strategies may differ. Implementing a comprehensive strategy that attends to one's mental and physical health is crucial for successfully navigating the difficulties associated with tinnitus.

The Effects Of Alcohol And Caffeine On Tinnitus

Tinnitus, a neurological disorder distinguished by the auditory perception of inaudible ringing, humming, or whistling in the ear canals, is susceptible to a range of environmental influences, including dietary decisions. Caffeine and alcohol, two frequently consumed substances, have been the subject of research regarding their prospective effects on tinnitus.

Caffeine, which is present in chocolate, coffee, tea, and energy beverages, has the potential to stimulate the central nervous system. There is some evidence to suggest that excessive caffeine consumption may worsen symptoms of tinnitus in certain individuals. The stimulant characteristics of caffeine have the potential to induce alterations in blood pressure and blood flow, which may have an impact on the auditory system. Nevertheless, the correlation between caffeine consumption and tinnitus is intricate and differs among individuals.

Individuals who are afflicted with tinnitus may challenge the effects of caffeine on their symptoms by reducing or eliminating their caffeine consumption. It is imperative to emphasize the potential significance of moderation, as sudden cessation of caffeine consumption may induce withdrawal symptoms and temporarily exacerbate tinnitus.

Additionally, alcohol, a depressant of the central nervous system, has been studied for tinnitus. Although certain studies have indicated a potential correlation between alcohol consumption and an elevated susceptibility to tinnitus, the available evidence remains inconclusive at best.

The potential impact of alcohol on blood flow in the auditory system is a subject of ongoing investigation. However, the precise correlation between alcohol and tinnitus has yet to be determined.

Alcohol consumption should be approached with moderation; individuals who suffer from tinnitus may benefit from monitoring their alcohol intake to determine whether or not it exacerbates their symptoms. Additionally, adequate hydration is crucial, as alcohol can exacerbate dehydration, a condition that may impact the severity of tinnitus.

In summary, the influence of caffeine and alcohol on tinnitus is a multifaceted and specific facet of the disorder. It is recommended that individuals diagnosed with tinnitus monitor their reactions to these substances and formulate well-informed judgments regarding their usage by their personal experiences.

CHAPTER THREE

Stress Reduction Strategies For The Management Of Tinnitus

A frequent contributor to the worsening of tinnitus symptoms is stress. Consequently, integrating stress reduction strategies into one's daily routine may prove to be a beneficial component in the management of tinnitus and the enhancement of general welfare.

A detrimental cycle may ensue when stress levels escalate, prompting an intensified consciousness of the tinnitus sounds; this, in turn, generates additional distress and further magnifies the perception of the sounds. As a result, it is critical to develop effective stress management techniques to disrupt this pattern.

Tinnitus can be mitigated and tension reduced through the use of a variety of techniques. Phenomena such as deep breathing exercises and mindfulness meditation are widely practiced to induce relaxation and divert attention from tinnitus symptoms. In addition to practicing yoga, spending time in nature, listening to soothing music, or participating in other activities that elicit feelings of pleasure and relaxation can all contribute to the alleviation of tension.

In addition to cognitive-behavioral therapy (CBT) and counseling, individuals who are experiencing the emotional effects of tinnitus may benefit from these interventions. The objective of these therapeutic approaches is to induce a more positive mindset by altering negative thought patterns and behaviors that are linked to tinnitus.

The integration of stress reduction strategies into one's daily routine constitutes a comprehensive strategy that not only aids in the management of tinnitus but also enhances one's mental and emotional state of being. Individuals with tinnitus must investigate various stress management techniques and determine which ones are most effective for them to develop an individualized plan.

Tracing The Relationship Between Tinnitus And Salt Consumption

The relationship between dietary choices, including salt intake, and tinnitus has been the subject of investigation. Certain findings indicate a possible correlation between elevated salt consumption and a worsening of tinnitus severity.

Salt overload may result in fluctuations in blood pressure, which may have adverse effects on the cardiovascular system. Tinnitus may be exacerbated by disturbances in the complex system of blood vessels within the ear, which are vulnerable to variations in blood flow. Certain studies posit that tinnitus symptoms might be alleviated by limiting sodium consumption, particularly in those who already have hypertension.

However, it is crucial to acknowledge that there is no consensus among scientists regarding the precise correlation between sodium and tinnitus. Certain studies have yielded inconclusive results regarding the relationship between sodium consumption and tinnitus, underscoring the necessity for additional research to elucidate the link.

Individuals who are afflicted with tinnitus may elect to follow a salt restriction plan to determine whether such a modification affects their symptoms. Adherence to a well-balanced diet and seeking guidance from healthcare professionals are recommended to verify the suitability of dietary modifications for one's overall health.

Analysis Of The Evidence Regarding The Relationship Between Sugar And Tinnitus

Considerable attention has been devoted to the potential effects of sugar consumption on a range of health conditions, tinnitus being one of them. Although the precise correlation between sucrose and tinnitus remains unknown, several studies indicate a plausible association that merits further investigation.

Elevated consumption of sugar has the potential to induce inflammation and oxidative stress, both of which have been linked to a range of health conditions, including those that influence the sense of hearing. Certain researchers posit that a decrease in sugar consumption could potentially serve as a modality to assuage tinnitus symptoms by mitigating inflammation.

Nonetheless, the evidence concerning the relationship between sucrose and tinnitus is inconclusive; further investigation is required to establish a definitive link. Furthermore, because individual reactions to dietary modifications may differ, those with tinnitus must monitor their own experiences and seek guidance from medical experts.

It is generally advised to uphold a balanced and healthful diet consisting of whole foods, fruits, vegetables, and restricted processed carbohydrates to promote overall well-being. Although there might be potential advantages to decreasing sugar consumption, individuals who have tinnitus must prioritize the evaluation of their comprehensive dietary regimen and rely on well-informed judgments that are specific to their situation.

Gluten And Tinnitus: Investigating The Possible Correlation

The protein gluten, which is present in wheat, barley, and rye, has generated considerable interest in the health community due to rumors surrounding its possible association with tinnitus. Certain individuals who have celiac disease, an autoimmune disorder precipitated by gluten ingestion, or gluten sensitivity have reported a correlation between gluten exposure and exacerbation of tinnitus symptoms.

The precise mechanisms that may underlie the possible association between gluten and tinnitus are still unknown. Certain hypotheses posit that inflammation and immune responses induced by gluten might play a role in the pathogenesis of tinnitus by disrupting the auditory system.

It is imperative to acknowledge that the available evidence concerning the correlation between gluten and tinnitus is restricted, and the omission of gluten from one's diet does not guarantee improvements for all individuals with tinnitus. Moreover, gluten intolerance and celiac disease are distinct medical conditions that necessitate expert medical diagnosis.

Those who have a suspicion regarding the potential correlation between gluten and their tinnitus may benefit from seeking guidance from healthcare experts, such as specialists in gastroenterology and otolaryngology, to investigate any possible underlying complications. Implementing a gluten-free diet without a correct diagnosis may not be appropriate for all individuals and should be performed with the supervision of medical professionals.

Further research is necessary to establish definitive associations and mechanisms about the potential correlation between gluten and tinnitus.

Gluten-sensitive individuals who experience tinnitus should consult a professional for assistance in establishing a precise diagnosis and developing effective management strategies.

CHAPTER FOUR

Tinnitus On The Mediterranean Diet

Tinnitus, which is distinguished by the involuntary perception of noise or ringing in the hearing, can be a difficult condition to control. Although a cure for tinnitus is currently absent, several lifestyle factors, such as one's nutrition, might be able to mitigate its symptoms. The Mediterranean Diet is a dietary approach that has garnered considerable attention in recent years due to its purported advantages.

The Mediterranean Diet encompasses more than mere weight loss; it embodies a way of life that mirrors the customary dietary conventions of nations situated along the Mediterranean Seashore. This nutritional regimen is abundant in whole cereals, fruits, vegetables, lean proteins, and healthy lipids, with particular emphasis on olive oil as the principal fat source. It is postulated that the fundamental elements comprising the Mediterranean Diet may exert a beneficial influence on general well-being and potentially offer distinct considerations in the context of tinnitus management.

An advantageous aspect of the Mediterranean Diet for those afflicted with tinnitus is its notable anti-inflammatory properties. It is believed that chronic inflammation is associated with a range of health conditions, tinnitus being one of them. The emphasis of the diet on omega-3 fatty acid-rich fruits, vegetables, and fatty salmon may aid in inflammation reduction. Moreover, tinnitus has been linked to oxidative stress; safeguarding against this condition may be the antioxidants found in these foods.

Moreover, there exists a correlation between the Mediterranean Diet and enhanced cardiovascular well-being. Tinnitus and cardiovascular problems are frequently associated; therefore, those who are experiencing tinnitus symptoms may indirectly benefit from this diet's promotion of heart health. A fiber-rich diet, consisting of legumes, seeds, and whole cereals, promotes cardiovascular health through the mitigation of cholesterol levels.

Although the Mediterranean Diet shows potential in the management of tinnitus, it is crucial to incorporate it into a comprehensive lifestyle transformation. Consistency in physical activity, proper hydration, and stress management are all equally essential elements. Furthermore, it is advisable for individuals suffering from tinnitus to seek guidance from a healthcare professional before implementing substantial dietary modifications. This will guarantee that the selected strategy is consistent with their holistic health requirements.

Tailored Tinnitus Dietary Strategies

Because every individual's body is distinct, personalized tinnitus diet plans have garnered attention as a potential solution to this condition's individualized characteristics. There are numerous potential underlying causes of tinnitus, and what is effective for one individual may not be so for another. Tailored tinnitus diet plans consider various components, including the individual's nutritional requirements, medical background, and pre-existing health conditions.

Developing a personalized tinnitus diet plan begins with a comprehensive evaluation of the patient's overall health. This includes determining whether culinary preferences may be affected by dietary restrictions, allergies, or sensitivities. In addition, it is critical to comprehend the individual's daily regimen and level of physical activity to develop a realistic and sustainable diet plan.

In dietary interventions for tinnitus, nutrient-dense foods that promote hearing health and reduce inflammation are frequently emphasized. An illustration of this would be the recommendation of vitamin B12-rich foods, including fish, meat, and dairy products, given the association between B12 deficiency and tinnitus. Individuals with tinnitus may also benefit from consuming magnesium-rich foods, such as almonds, seeds, and verdant green vegetables because magnesium has been shown to improve hearing function.

There may be instances where tinnitus sufferers are encouraged to consider implementing an elimination diet. This process entails methodically eliminating specific foods from the dietary regimen to identify potential irritants or triggers that may worsen symptoms of tinnitus. Frequently implicated substances encompass high-sodium foods, caffeine, and alcohol, albeit reactions may differ among individuals.

Monitoring and adjusting the personalized tinnitus diet plan regularly are also crucial to its success. A food diary is recommended for individuals to record their dietary consumption and monitor any fluctuations in tinnitus symptoms. After the observations of effects, this data may be utilized to optimize the diet regimen by eradicating or placing greater emphasis on particular foods.

Personalized tinnitus diet plans must be approached with a sense of patience and reasonable expectations. It may take some time for dietary modifications to produce perceptible results, and the objective is frequently not merely symptom relief but an improvement in overall health. Seeking advice from a healthcare professional, such as an otolaryngologist or registered dietitian, can offer significant assistance in developing an individualized tinnitus diet regimen that is to one's specific requirements and health objectives.

Observing Development And Modifying The Diet

The development of a tinnitus diet plan merely marks the beginning; consistent monitoring of progress and implementation of required modifications are essential components of tinnitus management via dietary interventions. Symptoms of tinnitus can be affected by a wide range of variables, and it may require some time for dietary modifications to produce discernible improvements.

A methodical and patient approach to monitoring is thus indispensable.

A comprehensive food diary serves as a pragmatic approach to monitoring dietary patterns and symptoms associated with tinnitus. The mealtimes and the quantities and varieties of foods consumed should be detailed in this journal. Additionally, throughout the day, individuals can record the frequency and severity of their tinnitus symptoms. Patterns may develop over some time, unveiling possible associations between specific food items and the worsening or alleviation of symptoms.

Consistent consultations with healthcare practitioners, such as otolaryngologists or dietitians, can yield significant knowledge. Experts can assist in analyzing the data gathered from the food diary and direct individuals in making well-informed modifications to their dietary regimens for tinnitus. Potential modifications could include substituting particular foods that appear to induce symptoms with more nutrients that promote auditory well-being.

Dietary modifications must be approached with extreme caution and implemented progressively. In some instances, abrupt dietary changes may result in unintended repercussions or nutritional imbalances. In addition, dietary modifications may require some time to become ingrained in the body; hastening the process could impede the ability to precisely evaluate their effect on tinnitus symptoms.

Apart from dietary considerations, there are additional lifestyle factors that individuals ought to be mindful of as they may have an impact on tinnitus. Stress, sleep deprivation, and excessive noise exposure are all potential contributors to tinnitus symptoms. By monitoring and addressing these factors in conjunction with dietary modifications, a more holistic strategy for tinnitus management can be achieved.

CHAPTER FIVE

Consulting Professionals For Guidance

It is crucial to consult a professional when considering dietary interventions for tinnitus to guarantee the implementation of safe and effective strategies. The etiology of tinnitus can be multifactorial, and a healthcare practitioner can assist in discerning the precise elements that contribute to an individual's manifestations. Seeking the expertise of an otolaryngologist, who specializes in the ear, nose, and throat, or a registered dietitian, can yield personalized recommendations that exceed the expectations of the individual.

A comprehensive assessment can be performed by an otolaryngologist to identify any potentially treatable medical conditions that may be the cause of tinnitus. Diagnostic procedures, including imaging studies and audiograms, might be suggested to evaluate the condition of the auditory system. After attending to any underlying medical concerns, the healthcare practitioner can engage in a collaborative effort with the patient to formulate an all-encompassing management strategy, which might encompass dietary suggestions.

Dietitians who are registered and possess specialized knowledge in the fields of audiology or otolaryngology can significantly contribute to the development of a diet regimen tailored to address tinnitus. They are capable of evaluating the nutritional requirements of an individual, taking into account any pre-existing health conditions, and offering recommendations grounded in empirical evidence. Furthermore, they possess the expertise to guide individuals through intricate dietary considerations, including remediating nutrient deficiencies and integrating particular nutrients that are recognized to promote auditory well-being.

Healthcare personnel may occasionally advise the use of complementary therapies in conjunction with dietary interventions. For individuals to contend with the psychological and emotional aspects of tinnitus, these may consist of cognitive-behavioral therapy, stress management techniques, or sound therapy.

Active participation in the management process and transparent communication with one's healthcare team are imperative for individuals diagnosed with tinnitus. By offering feedback regarding the efficacy of dietary modifications, disclosing any symptomatic changes, and engaging in discussions regarding concerns or obstacles, individuals can assist healthcare practitioners in formulating well-informed modifications to the treatment regimen.

In conclusion, collaboration with healthcare professionals is essential when investigating dietary strategies for the management of tinnitus to guarantee a safe and effective approach. In conjunction with a holistic evaluation of lifestyle elements, individualized dietary plans, consistent monitoring, and modifications can all contribute to a comprehensive management strategy for tinnitus sufferers.

Conclusion

In summary, although a definitive cure for tinnitus has yet to be established, mounting evidence indicates that dietary modifications might be utilized to alleviate its symptoms. The implementation of a tinnitus-friendly diet entails the reduction or elimination of specific substances that have the potential to worsen symptoms, including caffeine, alcohol, and nicotine.

Furthermore, the integration of anti-inflammatory foods, which are abundant in omega-3 fatty acids and antioxidants, could potentially alleviate the symptoms of tinnitus.

It is impossible to overstate the significance of sustaining overall health when it comes to tinnitus management. An inflammatory-reducing and immune-supporting diet that is well-balanced may have a beneficial effect on the severity of symptoms. It is essential to note, however, that individual responses to dietary modifications vary; what is effective for one person may not produce identical outcomes for another.

Additionally, before implementing substantial dietary modifications, it is imperative to seek guidance from a registered dietitian or a healthcare professional. They possess the ability to offer customized recommendations by an individual's health condition, thereby guaranteeing that dietary modifications are secure and individualized.

Fundamentally, although a tinnitus-specific diet may not provide an absolute remedy, it can serve as a beneficial element of a comprehensive strategy for coping with the condition.

By integrating dietary modifications with other lifestyle modifications and appropriate medical interventions, individuals who are seeking relief from tinnitus symptoms can develop a more comprehensive and efficacious approach to their condition.

THE END